T0016740

YOU KNOW YOU'RE A
GOLFER
WHEN...

HarperCollins*Publishers*

HarperCollins*Publishers*
1 London Bridge Street
London SE1 9GF

www.harpercollins.co.uk

HarperCollins*Publishers*
1st Floor, Watermarque Building, Ringsend Road
Dublin 4, Ireland

First published by HarperCollins*Publishers* 2022

10 9 8 7 6 5 4 3 2 1

Text by Tom Bromley © HarperCollins*Publishers* 2022
Illustrations by Ollie Man © HarperCollins*Publishers* 2022

HarperCollins*Publishers* asserts the moral right to be identified
as the author of this work

A catalogue record of this book is available from the British
Library

ISBN 978-0-00-850136-5

Printed and bound in the UK using 100% renewable electricity
at CPI Group (UK) Ltd

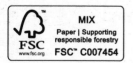

This book is produced from independently certified FSC™
paper to ensure responsible forest management.

For more information visit: www.harpercollins.co.uk/green

C🏌NTENTS

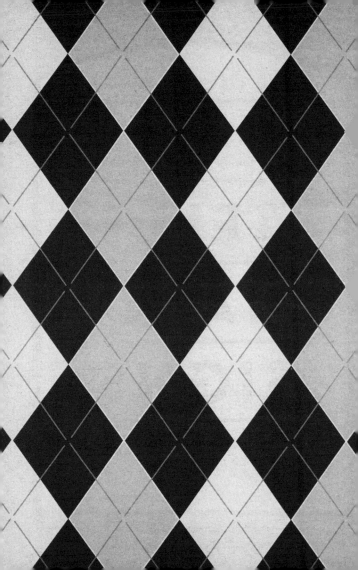

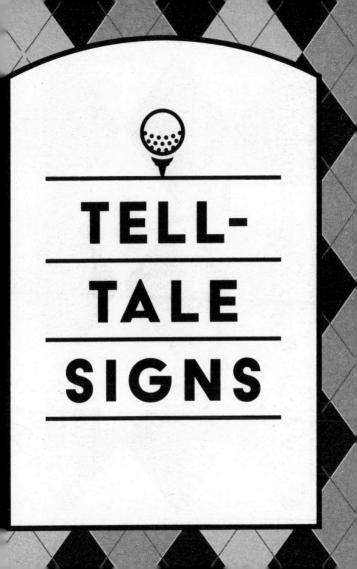

TELL-
TALE
SIGNS

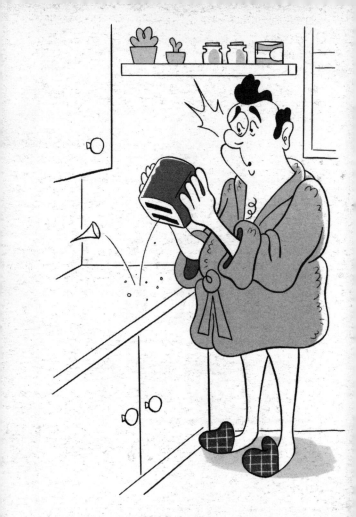

YOU FIND GOLF TEES IN THE ODDEST PLACES.

You frequently practise your swing with an imaginary club and ball, yet always look to see where it went.

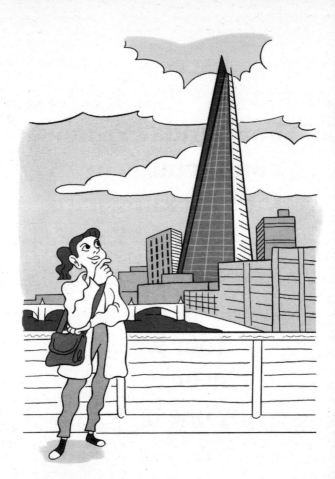

YOU'RE CONSTANTLY SIZING UP LANDMARKS TO DECIDE IF YOU COULD HIT OVER THEM WITH AN 8-IRON.

Your hands are most comfortable in an interlocking grip.

Your week can be ruined by one bogey.

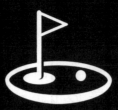

Your boss says you've been performing under par and you say, 'Thank you very much!'

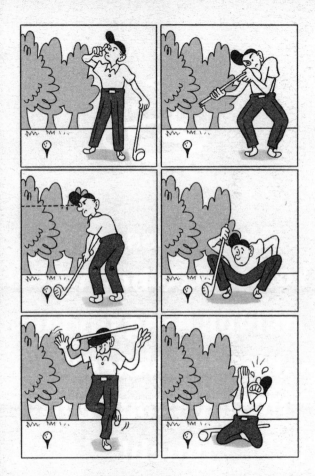

YOU HAVE A COMPLEX PRE-SHOT ROUTINE THAT YOU CAN'T DEVIATE FROM OR YOU KNOW YOUR BALL IS GOING STRAIGHT FOR THE ROUGH.

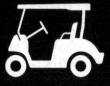

You take three times
as long as everyone
else to take their
putt at crazy golf.

You're buying a new car
and your main concern is
whether your golf clubs
will fit.

The drive of your life
doesn't involve a Ferrari
or a Porsche.

Your most searched terms
on Google are 'golf' and
'weather'.

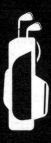

You believe that
ultimate authority
lies not with
the government,
but with the R&A.

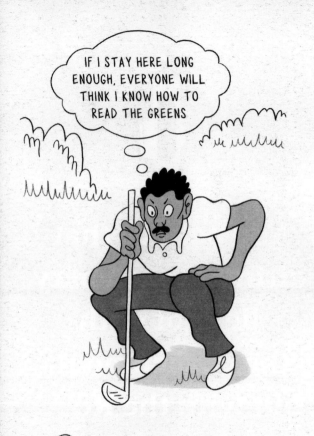

YOU KNOW HOW TO ACT THE PART.

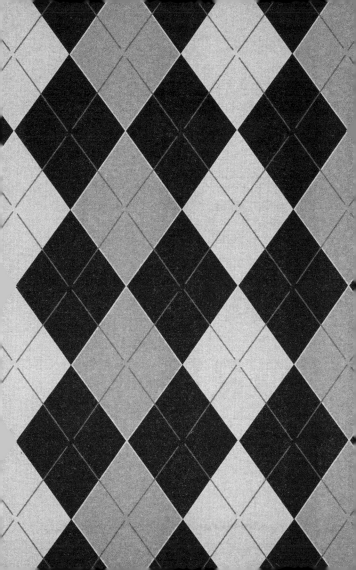

FOOD AND DRINK

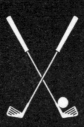

You like a club
sandwich for lunch
(preferably with
chips).

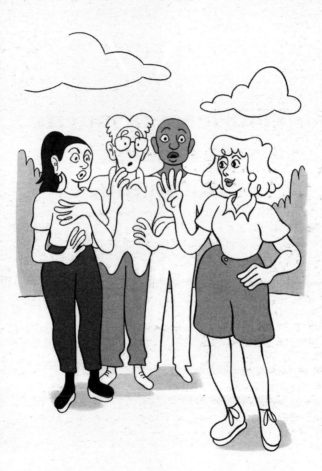

**YOU DON'T HAVE ANY QUALMS ABOUT
SUGGESTING A FOURSOME.**

**Your least favourite
cut of meat is
the shank.**

You've tried
the golfing diet
of greens and water.

You disagree
with the dietician
that roughage is
good for you.

You're always thirsty as you have an aversion to water.

You eat pizza in portions rather than slices.

You hear, 'Don't drink and drive' and think, 'Good advice, I'd slice it horribly after two pints.'

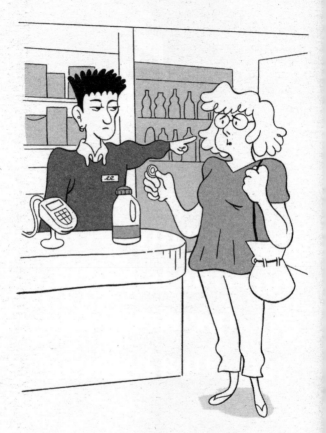

**YOU'VE TRIED TO BUY A PINT OF MILK
WITH A BALL MARKER.**

**Your favourite
wine is claret
(preferably
in a jug).**

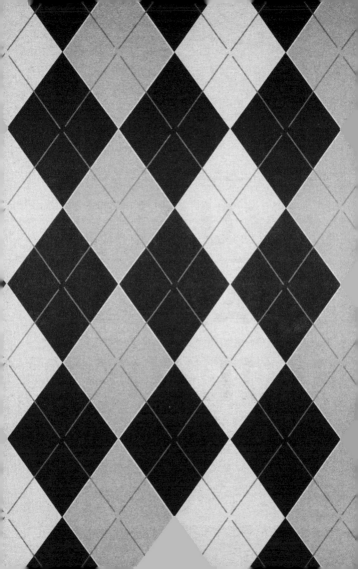

MUSIC
AND
CULTURE

Your favourite band is the Eagles.

You're the only person who doesn't groan when the Birdie Song comes on.

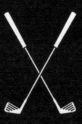

You hear 'Gimme!
Gimme! Gimme!'
by Abba and
immediately think
of that chip shot you
hit to six inches.

You understand why Michael Jackson only wore one glove.

People talk about the King and you think of Arnold Palmer rather than Elvis.

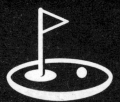

You hear the
Pearl & Dean music
at the cinema
('Par par par par
par par ...') and
think of Nick Faldo's
final round at
Muirfield in 1987.

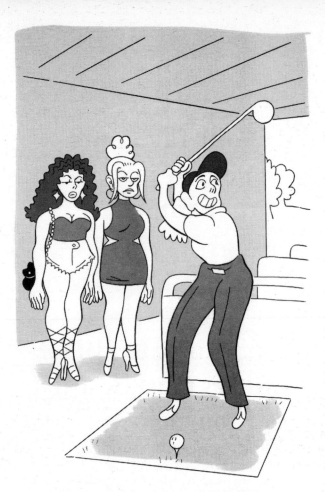

**YOUR IDEA OF NIGHTCLUBBING IS AN
EVENING AT THE DRIVING RANGE.**

Your favourite sort of joke is azinger.

You assume the Dutch Masters must be a golf tournament.

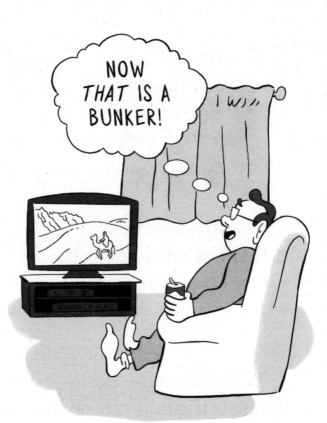

YOU DON'T HAVE A TRUE MOVIE CONNOISSEUR'S APPRECIATION OF *LAWRENCE OF ARABIA*.

You can quote
Caddyshack
line by line.

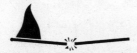

**Your favourite
Marvel character is
Iron Man.**

Your favourite Bond
scene is the golf match in
Goldfinger.

You think Fungus
the Bogeyman
should probably
have worked on his
putting a bit more.

Your 'luxury item' for *Desert Island Discs* would be a sand wedge.

Your swing rehearsal would put Michael Flatley to shame.

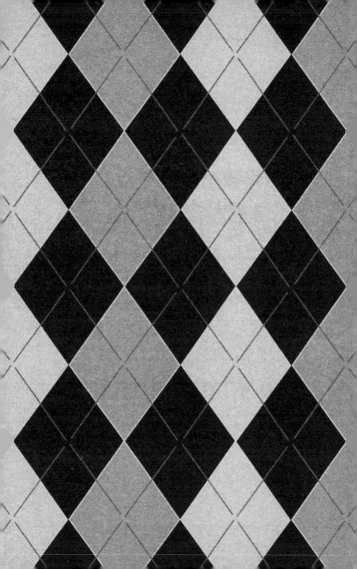

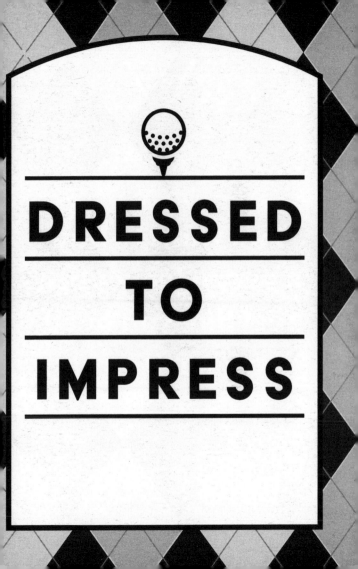

DRESSED

TO

IMPRESS

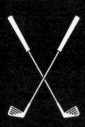

You want to buy
a green jacket but
feel like you need
to earn it first.

You adjust your golf cap even when you're not wearing one.

You always tuck your shirt in.

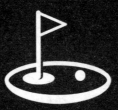

You turn down
the offer of some
Pringles, smugly
thinking that golfing
fashion has moved
on since then.

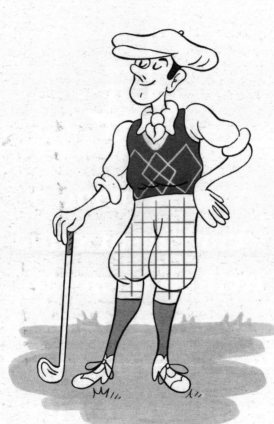

**YOU DON'T THINK THIS OUTFIT LOOKS
ENTIRELY RIDICULOUS.**

You start a
conversation
with a complete
stranger just
because they're
wearing a golf hat.

You wear two pairs of socks in case you get a hole in one.

You wear gloves in your back pocket more often than on your hands.

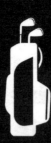

You instinctively try to tip your cap when you see someone you know, even if you aren't wearing a cap.

Your most expensive item of clothing is your golf shoes.

You own at least one golf cap.

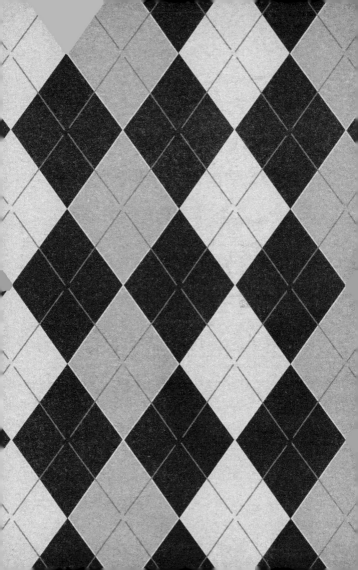

HOLIDAYS

AND

SPECIAL

OCCASIONS

**You think
St Andrews
would be a great
destination for a
family holiday.**

You celebrate special
occasions by playing
36 holes.

You don't always
carry a spare tyre
but you always
have an emergency
golf club.

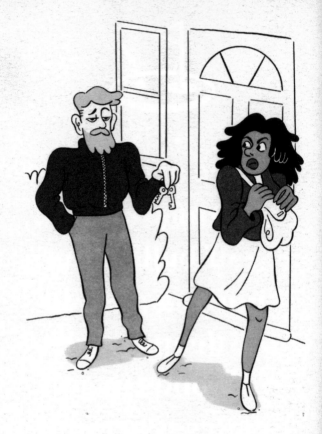

YOU'RE ON A DAY OUT AND YOU WON'T LET
YOUR PARTNER PUT ANYTHING IN YOUR BAG,
EXPLAINING SHARING IS AGAINST CLUB
REGULATIONS.

There are at least 100 of your old golf balls lying underwater/in the deep roughs/ in woods in golf courses around the country.

You keep coins from foreign holidays to use as markers.

You have a tell-tale golf tan of bronzed arms and pale hands.

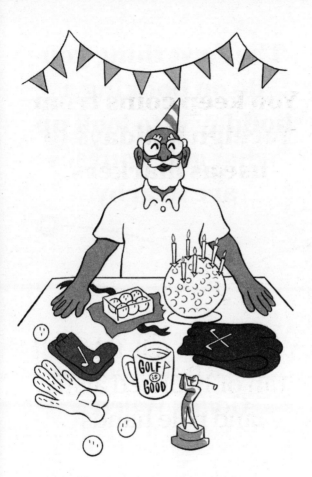

EVERYONE BUYS YOU GOLF-RELATED PRESENTS FOR YOUR BIRTHDAY.

The first thing you do on booking a holiday is to look up what golf courses are nearby.

You own a book called *You Know You're a Golfer When ...*

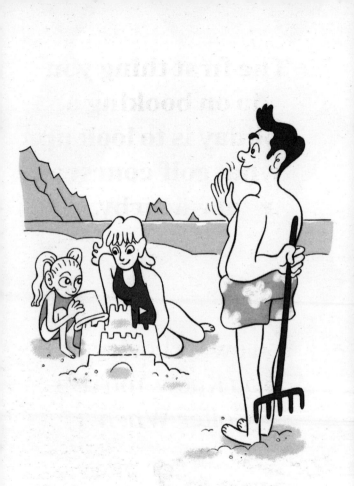

YOU GO FOR A WALK ON THE BEACH AND HAVE THE URGE TO GET A RAKE OUT.

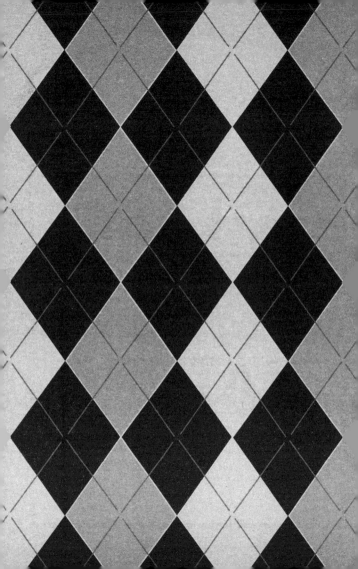

GOLFERS
VS
NATURE

**Your favourite
animal is a tiger.**

Your least favourite
animal is a cheetah.

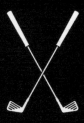

Your favourite
kind of dog is
a big dog.

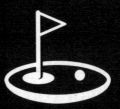

You like to pluck
a few blades of
grass and watch
them fall, just to
see which way
the wind blows.

You can't go on a walk
without replacing every
divot you see.

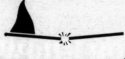

**You wear your golf shoes
on a hike.**

You know a walk is a round
of golf spoiled.

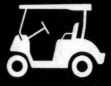

You know
the truth about
trees: that
they're at least
90 per cent air.

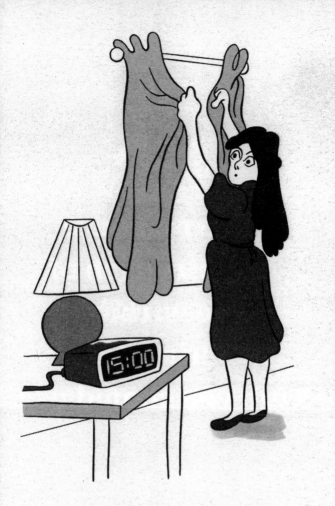

YOU THINK TWILIGHT IS FROM 3 P.M.

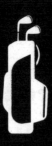

You measure
the strength of
the wind by
debating which
club you should use.

**You consider
a round of golf
great exercise.**

You go for a walk
in a forest and
think, 'Hazard'.

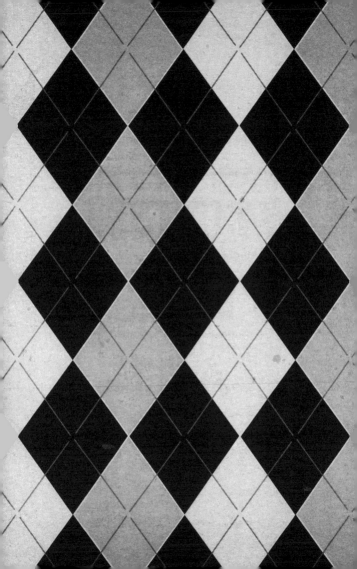

MORE TELL-TALE SIGNS

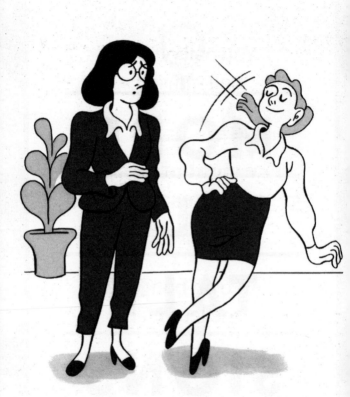

**YOU DON'T KNOW HOW TO STAND STILL
IF YOU'RE NOT LEANING ON A CLUB.**

You call pennies
'ball markers'.

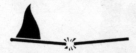

**The sight of smooth
grass makes you drool.**

You're on board with
the leaf rule.

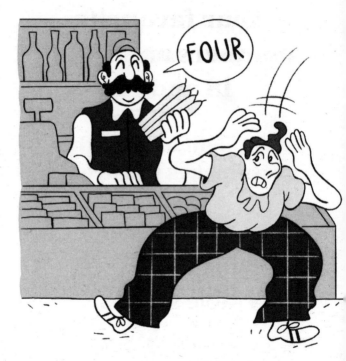

YOU CAN'T HEAR THE WORD 'FOUR' WITHOUT IMMEDIATELY PROTECTING YOUR HEAD.

Your favourite numbers are 2, 3, 4, 18 and 72.

You wonder what a snooker table stimps.

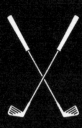

You're distracted at a funeral, thinking what a nice golf course the cemetery would have made.

You spontaneously feel the urge to spread your legs and wiggle your bottom.

You find yourself discussing your shaft loudly in public.

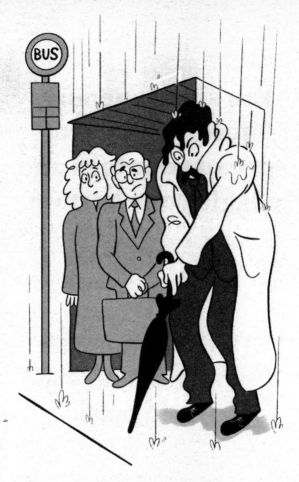

YOU CAN'T HOLD A COLLAPSED LONG
UMBRELLA WITHOUT PRACTISING YOUR SWING.

You would have
no concerns
about proposing a
threesome to your
partner.

Someone asks if you believe in miracles and you reply, 'Medinah'.

You prefer to pay via chip and pin.

You start looking
forward to your
Saturday round
by lunchtime on
Monday.

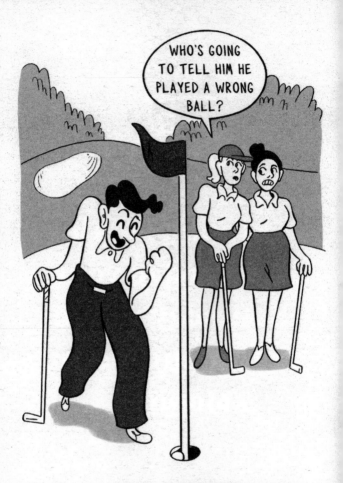

YOUR WORST NIGHTMARE DOESN'T INVOLVE VAMPIRES OR MURDERERS.

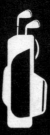

You rate your friends based on their availability for a round and how likely you are to beat them.

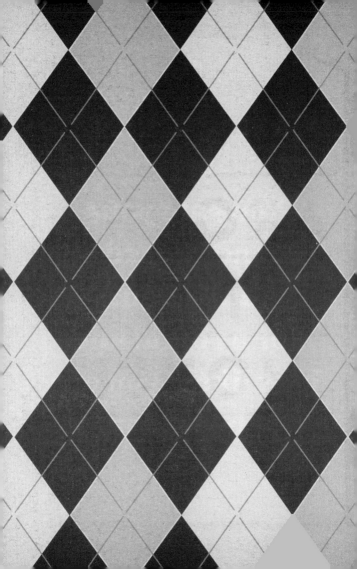

AROUND THE HOUSE

Your dream house is on the edge of a golf course.

You've broken at least one ornament from practising your swing in the house.

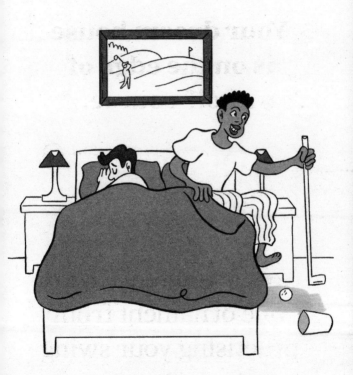

**YOU HAVE A BALL, A PUTTER AND
A BEAKER IN THE BEDROOM FOR
SOME LATE-NIGHT PUTTING PRACTICE.**

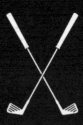

Your partner
asks you to buy
a new iron and
you come back with
a Callaway Apex.

You won't share your tea caddy with anyone else.

You've practised teeing your ball up at home so you look good on the course.

You see leaves and twigs in the yard and think, 'What a lot of loose impediment!'

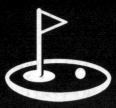

You've looked
at your child's
favourite soft toy
and wondered if
it would make a
good cover for your
clubs when they
grow out of it.

You set up the bedroom mirror so you can watch how you swing.

You have your own golf towel, rather than stealing one from the bathroom.

You've debated giving your son a middle name of Seve or Tiger.

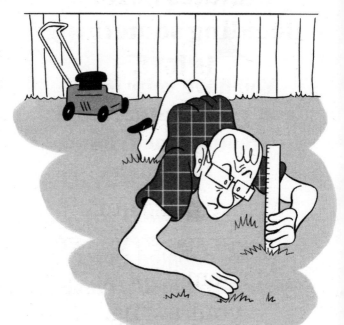

YOU MOW YOUR LAWN TO FAIRWAY HEIGHT.

You'll never search for more than five minutes before deciding something is lost.

You've rearranged the garage so you've got room to practise your swing.

You ask the greenkeeper for advice on how to turn your garden into a putting green.

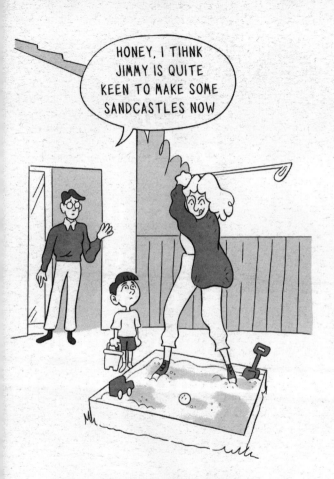

YOU FIND ANY OCCASION TO
PRACTISE YOUR SWING.

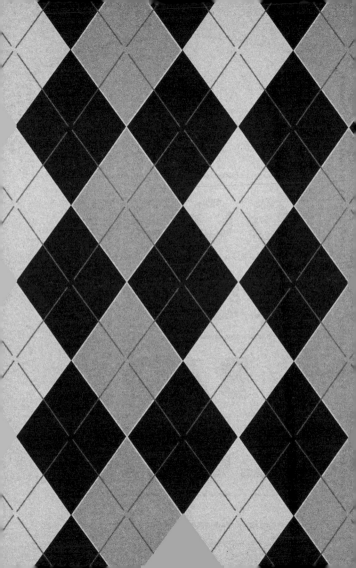

GOOD LUCK, BAD LUCK

You have thrown
a club in frustration
after a bad shot.

**You've had at least one
bout of the yips.**

A bad round ruins
your entire week.

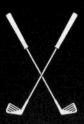

You haven't
successfully
performed your
trick shot for 15
years, yet still talk
about it every time
you play.

You're completely convinced you're better than your handicap would suggest.

You know you've hit the putt wide the moment you've touched the ball.

You wake up at night in a cold sweat, thinking about that putt you missed five years ago.

You have at least one
good-luck charm on
your golf bag.

You've blamed your
club for the shot
you've just hit.

You've cursed
the person who
designed the course
you're playing on.

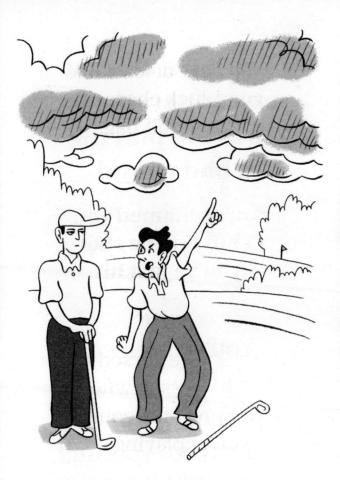

**YOU'VE BLAMED THE SUN IN YOUR
EYES FOR A BAD SHOT.**

You have at least one superstition to avoid playing a bad round.

You've blamed everything possible for a bad round ... apart from yourself.

You've sworn after a bad round you'll never play this stupid game again, yet are back on the course the following weekend.

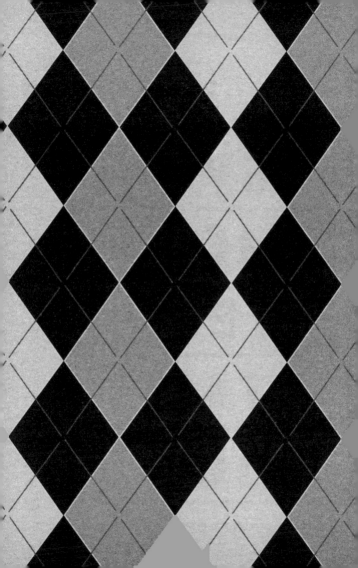

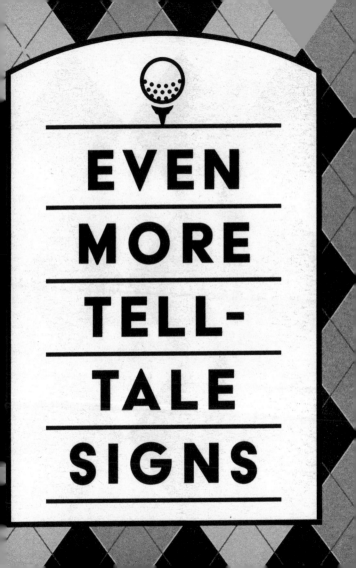

EVEN
MORE
TELL-
TALE
SIGNS

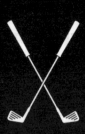

You can't get out of
bed to go to work,
but rise and shine
at 6 a.m. at
the weekend for
your round.

You wonder whether winter rules can be extended into March. And April. And May ...

You don't blush when telling someone you need to wash your balls.

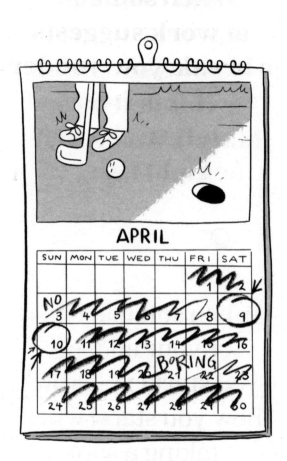

THE SECOND WEEKEND IN APRIL IS SACRED.

**When someone
at work suggests
a break, you wonder
if it is from
left to right,
or right to left ...**

When someone asks
for your address,
you start explaining
how you stand when
taking a shot.

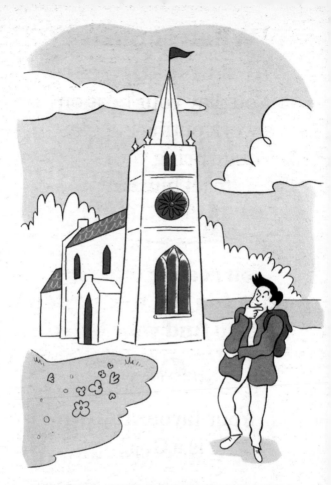

YOU SEE A FLAG ON TOP OF A BUILDING AND THINK, 'I'VE SEEN SOME DIFFICULT PIN PLACEMENTS BEFORE ...'

You play your boss on
a work outing but can't
quite bring yourself
to let him win.

You realise that the
older you get, the harder
it is to find your balls.

Your favourite car
is a Golf.

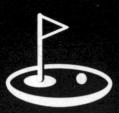

You arrive early at
the course to warm
up your swing
before your round
(and still shank your
opening drive).

You judge a garden by the smoothness of the grass.

You never break the speed limit as you don't like going over 70.

You keep a set of golf clubs in the boot of the car, because you never know ...

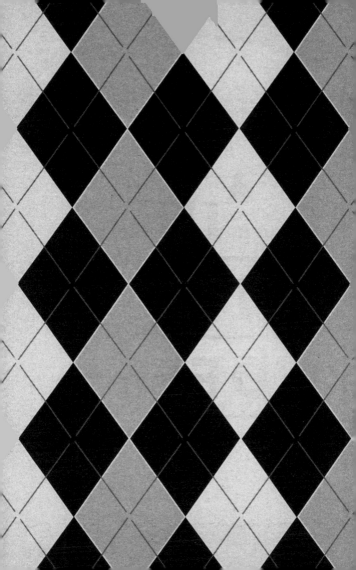

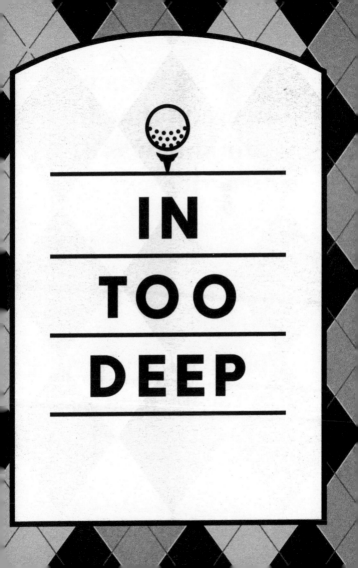

IN
TOO
DEEP

You no longer pretend that an air shot was a practice swing.

You no longer have first-tee jitters.

You've spent a lot more money than you can afford on gadgets that have not helped your game at all.

You pick up
the tee before
the ball lands.

**You have your own
divot tool.**

The clubs in your bag
no longer match.

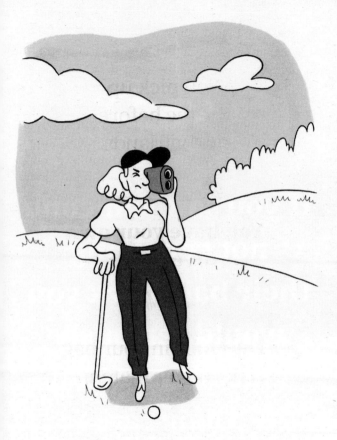

YOU CAN SPEND UP TO SIX MINUTES WORKING OUT IF THE HOLE IS 178 OR 179 YARDS AWAY.

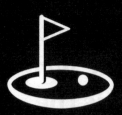

If you saw someone
not repairing
their ball mark you
would seriously
consider keying
their car.

You think picking up the wrong golf ball is the eighth deadly sin.

You know what the coefficient of restitution is.

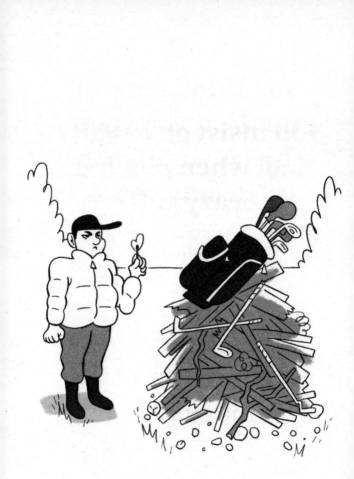

A BAD DAY FOR YOU IS MUCH MORE EXPENSIVE THAN ANYONE ELSE'S BAD DAY.

You insist on a white ball when playing crazy golf.

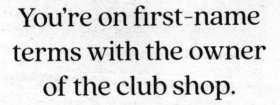

You're on first-name terms with the owner of the club shop.

You stop to talk
to someone in
a hallway and
automatically
start practising
your swing.

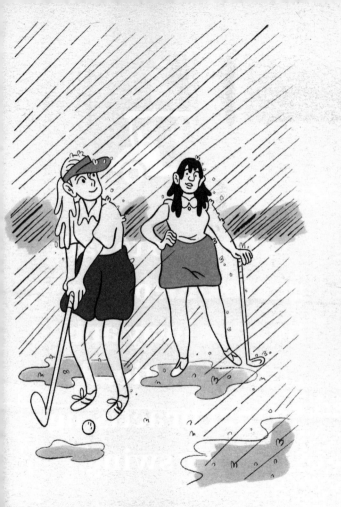

NOTHING DAMPENS YOUR SPIRIT.

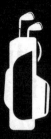

When you finally
get to death's door,
heaven looks a hell
of a lot like your
favourite fairway.

**Everyone in front of
you is slow
and everyone
behind you is fast.**

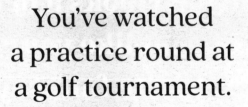

You've watched
a practice round at
a golf tournament.

You keep checking
your phone on
the day the Ryder
Cup wildcards
are announced ...
just in case.